Dedicated to:

....

From:...........................

Date...........................

Note...........................

....

....

....

....

....

MY SON, what every child with Autism wants you to know

MY SON, WHAT EVERY CHILD WITH AUTISM WANTS YOU TO KNOW
BY SILVANA ARMENTANO PEREZ
THIS IS A PRODUCTION OF MUSIK HOPE
P.O. BOX 266174
WESTON FLORIDA 33326
WWW.SILVANAARMENTANO.COM

PUBLISHED BY MUSIK HOPE
ID: LE 1030 PAPERBACK
ISBN: 9781980837237   PAPERBACK
FIRST EDITION 2018
CATEGORY: FAMILY / RELATIONSHIPS / NON-FICTION / EDUCATION

WRITTEN AND REVIEWED BY SILVANA ARMENTANO
DESIGN COVER SILVANA ARMENTANO
COPYRIGHT © 2018 BY SILVANA ARMENTANO PEREZ
ALL INTERNATIONAL RIGHTS RESERVED

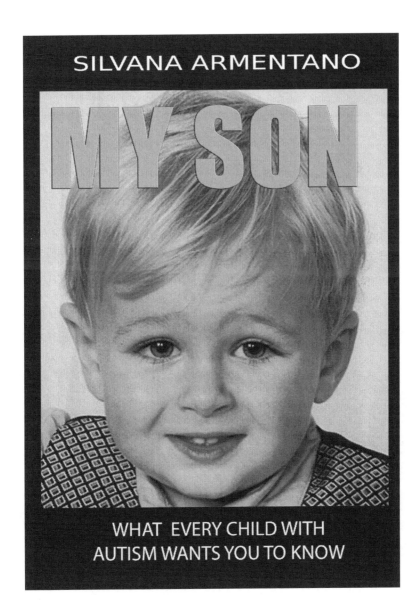

Silvana, God has crowned my life with you, my only woman and my only wife, my love. I know that through the pages of this book, I have acquired wisdom to live wisely with you and with David. We have a solid and firm home that we have formed together and is founded on the rock, our Lord Jesus Christ. I wish and declare that the understanding of many people will read this book will be opened their minds with this profound book that God inspired you and you will touch millions of people with your teachings. Keep moving forward, I bless you, support and admire you. Your husband who loves you.

Dr. Daniel Perez

Dear Mom, you are my Angel, Thank you for being my Mom. I love you

David John Perez your son.

Table of Content

YOU CAN DEFEAT AUTISM!

Keep reading until the end

Introduction

I have seen depressed and destroyed people, discovering that their baby is affected by autism and other child syndromes. If you are distressed, in denial or just want to learn to understand what autism it is, and how you can help your child to progress in life, I invite you to read with me throughout the entire book and I will teach you ten important things that every child with Autism wants you to know.

Through many years of experience teaching music to children with all kinds of talents and medical situations, I went through many opportunities of learning, experiences of all kinds and achieved strategies that helped me to get ahead. These experiences and tips I want to share with you and promote your children to the highest possible level.

There were situations that even I thought that God was not fair and he had forgotten about me and my family. But now I learned that my life would have been not the same without my little angel David. My son's name is David and we are working together to defeat this neurological disorder called autism.

MY SON, what every child with Autism wants you to know

My son taught me real meaning of the true love, without words or glances. He gave a special meaning to my life and it is or more beautiful and beautiful that God could have given me. I was chosen among many women as the best and only qualified for this mission possible. I was selected from the specialized squad of great challenges and my beloved son gave me the opportunity to grow and to love unconditionally. I want you to also feel this for your son, and that everything that is overwhelming you now disappears and you think there is a way out and hope.

This book was born with the idea that I could help people get up and understand that having a child with a medical condition is not a bad thing to die. Turn pain into a gift and see the smile of many children and families a reality is the purpose of this book.

In my long journey through helping my son David, I saw many parents also are able to give away their own children just because they have autism or some physical defects. That's cruel? Many other parents think they are not normal, others who are sick.

But STOP! All children are special and perfect according to the lens you use to see them. So much cruelty only promotes bad things in the world. Our children are worth than gold, our children are not sick, our children are normal. Our children are capable of doing what a child who does not have autism can do, if you believe it.

Your son is the best thing that has happened to you in your entire life. That their abilities are momentarily affected by the infantile syndrome of autism or other medical situations, He or she are still unique and perfect, special and a human being who needs help to be and function in a society demanding and perfectionist as we live today.

Have I not commanded you? Be strong and courageous. Do not be frightened, and do not be dismayed, for the Lord your God is with you wherever you go. This phrase full of faith and courage has always accompanied me throughout my long journey with autism. My dear friends, do not get tired, do not get depressed, do not fall, do not get to deny your little one to ignore or reject him. He is a human being and deserves the same opportunity as others. Always try to give him the life's dignity he deserves, to help him make progress and overcome

MY SON, what every child with Autism wants you to know

autism. Because something that you can achieve as a parent is to help overcome the autism that is affecting your child. It's time for you to be brave for your son, and face the world and change your mind.

The challenges that life presents to you are opportunities to grow, take advantage of them. What you sow today you will reap it up tomorrow and you will sleep in peace of having given the maximum of your resources and strengths and to have removed your beloved son from autism spectrum disorder, that will be your maximum prize in life. Be Strong! you're not alone,

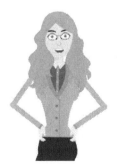 I understand you. With God's help, who does not abandon us, and the advice of this book and professionals, you will be the best father or mother your son can have.

YOU CAN OVERCOME AUTISM!

Silvana Armentano

1. I want you to know ... 10 Things I do without control

"... Mom, I want you to know that I love you and I need your help. Mommy I have no control of my body and sometimes I move a lot because I do not feel my body in the space. Could you help me feel my body correctly? Do not get mad at me please, I'm not in control of that and I'm too small to fix it by myself. "I want to see you happy, do we fix together this mess?

Realizing that your child is a child with symptoms of autism and accept this true as it is, is a strong process that as parents is difficult to overcome.

Children affected by autism spectrum disorder almost always from babies give signs that their health could be affected with this condition.

As parents and human beings that we are, it is hard for us to realize and accept it. Although they are small signs, these are enough to go to the doctor and look for a diagnosis and put together an immediate action plan.

MY SON, what every child with Autism wants you to know

Accept your child and love him as he is!

It is not good or nice to say, that your child is not normal, or that you refuse to see the reality of his health for fear of what the people around you will say or the challenges that will come upon you.

Always loves your son very much, because it is a gift that not everyone can have. If you notice that your child does not use the toys as other appropriately babies use, Example: He always takes the carts to his mouth, while his friends roll them on the floor, and your son always tends to get away from the other children, that is a clear signal that you must pay attention.

Parents! do not get scared when you notice these signs, rather this signs should motivate you to seek immediate professional and appropriate help for your child. Autism is a neurological disorder, a condition that must be treated as soon as possible.

Do not delay to visit the doctor a do an evaluation and waist your time and waist your child's life to wait for more signs and more signs, with about three signs is enough reason to go to a specialist. Do not expect to start helping your child when he starts school and it is already very big, and you can already see a very remarkable difference in his development. As early as you start helping him, better and more opportunities he will have and his quality of life will be better and he will get out of this medical situation faster than you can imagine.

The main idea is to attend and provide all help possible to the needs of your child as soon as possible; from Baby age, and to provide all professional help and minimize the limitations that cause autism in children and maximize opportunities to overcome autism.

I will give you 10 very generalized and alarming autism's signs, which are noticed in children at early age who are affected by their abilities by this neurological disorder called autism. If you have already seen these signs in your child, then do not wait any longer and seek professional help, there is no time to lose. He needs you and you are the most important person in the world who can do it. That is your privilege to help your children succeed.

Clear signs of autism

1. He doesn't look to your eyes.

MY SON, what every child with Autism wants you to know

This childhood syndrome called autism affects social relationships and the child does not usually look into the eyes to establish visual communication with others. They tend to look more at the mouth or in space when we talk to them. The eye contact is poor or does not exist. It seems that they are not listening or as if they were in another world. If you notice that your little one, always has the lost eye contact, this could be a sign. Forward I will give solutions and ideas to activate eye contact.

2. Does not respond to his name.

If your son is more than 12 months, and you call him by his name and does not turns his head to look at you, it is a signal that you should pay close attention and there could be some signs of autism. The lack of social attention, is one of the main challenges that a special child faces daily. This signal, which does not respond to its name when they call it and seems an apparent deafness, within the autistic spectrum, this could be an important sign and it appeared at an early age, from baby.

3. Inappropriate play.

My personal experience of dealing with autism at home and with some of my students has taught me that inappropriate play may be another important feature to detect autism at an early age. My son always used toys in a strange way. If it was a telephone, He used it to hammer the floor. If it was a CD He used it as a top spin. If it was a car, he would focus on looking at the wheels and bringing it to his mouth. If you consider that your child is old enough to use the toys correctly and understand their functionality, and you see that he has not yet doing that, it could be a signal to detect autism.4.

4. Poor Social Interaction Analyzing the name of the "Autism" syndrome, morphologically it contains "Auto" which in Greek means "by itself". The child may seem very introverted or in his own world. Social relations are not of his interest. The child who presents these signs creates a self-sufficient and self-stimulating world where it is not necessary needed to have relationships with people. He only comes closer and interacts when he needs something, for example: food

5. Stereotyped repetitive movements They tend to make movements like tics very quickly and without meaning.

For example, he can sit quietly for many hours in the preferred chair, doing the same thing over and over again, moving his arms like wings clapping or making sounds.

6. They walk on tiptoe. There are many reasons why children with autistic signs walk on their tiptoes. The vast majority of parents think that their little one has developed a very sophisticated walk, but the truth is that children find it easier to walk on their tiptoes. They are looking for pressure on their feet because they probably they do not feel their body in space and they need to stimulate their body to feel it.

7. They lose expressive language or speech does not exist. Children who exhibit these autistic signs usually use very few words or sounds. They have trouble forming complete sentences or having a conversation. The pronunciation of the words is very difficult for them and sometimes you do not understand what they are saying.

The verbal communication that most often use are repetitive sounds isolated words or abstract signs, that you as a parent must have all the patience in the world to learn to understand and respond to them. You must have love for your child, the more patience and technique you have better communication with them. I will give more examples later.

8. They do not feel pain.

It is not that they do not feel pain, but that they do not know how to react to it. Autism affects the sensory functions causing a disorder in the correct reaction of the five senses, taste, touch, smell, hearing, vision. That's why they do not feel the pain or do not respond to his name. If your baby falls and he does not cry or cry very little, you should immediately consult this with a doctor. This is the easiest signal to detect in children, they always have accidents and falls.

9. Bad sleep, bad digestion. The selectivity at the time of eating, the repulsion to certain foods, tantrums, constant vomiting, could be an important sign to consider. They are sensitive to the varied textures of foods. On the other hand, their sleeping habits are very inconstant. The child may not have slept all day, and when he falls asleep, he wakes up after a maximum of 20 minutes and resists awake the entire day.

10. Development Delay. Every process of learning by imitation will become more difficult. Teach him to go to the bathroom, to give smiles, how to socialize, to draw, to drink water from a cup, to eat by itself, it will take a little more time and training. My neighbor gave birth almost at the same time as me, and it was obvious how her little daughter was developing her attitudes and aptitudes, and my David did not even say hello.

Do not worry, if you realize that your child has some of these sign of autism, God's plan is still perfect for everyone. Take care of him, love him as he is right now, give him love, educate him and help him. Give your child everything he needs to overcome and defeats autism and never make him feel rejection. You cannot win a battle without fighting it.

Yes, YOU CAN Defeat AUTISM!

Read up to the end!

2. I want you to know ... I want to tell you something but you do not understand me

"... I am so excited to tell my entire family that I love them, but my body does not respond. I can listen to what my family say about me and understand that something happens to me that sadden them and they do not understand, that's why I get apart and alone. I am a member of the Family and I accept the rest as they are Can they accept me and love me as I am too? I am a member of the family and I cannot do anything to get the autism out of me Could you please help me? United, We can more. I need them..."

It is not easy to talk about special people, when you refer to your own child or a family member. The first time you thought about it, your hands got cold, the second, and the third ... and you're still learning. If your child or family member has siblings, then it is not the only special; all members are special. They are a beautiful special family; God chose you for this Great Mission and you are truly fortunate!

MY SON, what every child with Autism wants you to know

In your daily life routine, there are innumerable challenges and become an extreme test for everyone to integrate your child and your family into normal social life activities outside of the home. Integrating your child to our community outside the comfort of your home to simple activities such as going to the supermarket, a social event, a birthday, going to church or a festive celebration requires an admirable effort that are a very challenging and stressful. In the process of the activity, our behavior, has to be what is socially acceptable and appropriate and autism makes more difficult our daily routines.

Integration is synonymous with inclusion; we generally use these terms lightly, only referring to the addition or addition of someone or something to a set. We associate it with words such as: introduce, encompass, incorporate, insert, attach, frame, wrap, encompass; the reality is that inclusion includes more profound aspects. When we include we are recognizing that we all have different skills, characteristics and potential as well as needs. We all have the right to be, "part of" the community.

On the other hand, we have the exclusion, antonym of all the above. Separate or eliminate the individual or thing from the group. In the case of special families, it is to separate our child from the typical social life and routine activities. Due to the health condition and because we work differently than a typical normal family we limit ourselves and deprive in all or some areas outside and inside our house. All the activities of a child or special adult are functional according to their health or behavior.

There is fear, looks, restrictions, disqualifications, omissions. We deprive ourselves to do many things and activities. We lock ourselves or hide from others for what they will say. Usually we hide our way of special and particular living because of social rejection and we suffer the pain of loneliness and not being part of what "normal" people are accustomed. Love is the best communication and tool. Love covers a multitude of faults.

Get organized! It's the key. Do not be afraid of what others will say, do not be afraid of being different and original, or afraid of the rejection because of the behavior of our children and relatives. Being different is not something to be ashamed of. You have to make important decisions, always thinking what is best for you; do not think about the comfort of others. God created us all: we are unique, different, special; God created the earth to share it and enjoy life with all communities. No two individuals are the same, we all have different abilities to share and that are the wonderful differences that should never stop us from astonishing and reinforce.

If your family is special as mine, it is because God chose you with love and compassion as an instrument for a great mission. They are families that knows the value of a simple smile, compassionate, patient; they will know how to act and control the situations that will be presented to them. We are a fortunate family. We are different and that enriches us.

Get up! I want you not to be intimidated or hurt by the standards of being different or normal. Be creative and original in everything you do. Be happy at all times and at all places, every day. Enjoy the challenges of including your entire family in all activities and events that are presented to you daily; Also including those who have special needs is not an easy task, but possible. Breathe deeply; be courageous, calm, strong and face the community challenges with love every time is necessary. Baby Step by baby step, without haste but without stopping; putting a grain of sand each time, life will run its course. Everything will be possible with effort, faith perseverance and dedication. You will win and you will succeed in this mission. You are not alone; you are not alone.

An activity that will help you start being included can be the following: Go to your neighbor's birthday party, the whole family for a lapse of 15 minutes.

I will propose the following suggestions:

1. Set short and small goals; One step at a time, first you have to walk before you learn to run.

2. Be proud of the achievement of leaving the comfort zone. Be happy not to be afraid or ashamed to be ridiculed at some point. Try it until you achieve it, love, faith and strategies for short periods.

3. Congratulate your special family member for deciding to accept and collaborate in this mission, leaving the comfort of their safe environment. He also tried hard because he has trouble doing some things.

4. Have an emotional support plan for any unexpected circumstances that could come up. There will be periods of time with nothing to do; Take games and toys with you to occupy your child with appropriates activities. Be brave, you already are embarked on the trip.

5. Avoid listening to negative comments about the behavior of your special family member, especially criticism. Prepare to talk about autism, break the silence; respond and talk with people who value what you have achieved and are interested in listening to you. You are the specialist of your child's condition and the one who will advocate for them best against anyone or any situation.

6. Repeat the experience for a longer period of time. Already your family member and your entire family knows what to expect from the family reunion. They are ready for a little while more. Be patient and kind at all times.

7. Plan new adventures, activities and different and enjoyable events to attend or perform. Write them down in an agenda. Enjoy all the short time. Better short and good times than long and bad times.

8. Share to other family members the dreams and plans you hope to achieve for the near future. Your family support is essential for this mission of including your special family member in a family life routine inside and outside the home. Together and united your team can achieve it.

9. Focus on the achievements obtained during the entire process of the activity since it was planned, when you communicated it to the whole family and when you told your special family member. Everything counts. What they enjoyed in the process and what they did well in the activity. Celebrate what went well and analyze how to improve the rest. Progress does not have to be absolute or perfect.

10. Trust in God, put all your faith in Him. Ask Him for you, your special family member and all the other members of your family. They will be able to integrate their family to the typical daily activities of society little by little, one day at a time.

Yes, YOU CAN Defeat AUTISM!

Read up to the end!

SONG FOR MY SON, MY SON

Music And Lyrics : Copyright © Silvana Armentano

My son, how much you've grown
I still can feel you kicks in my womb.
Today quite a men full of dream.
You have everything to conquer and achieve.

Everything you touch prospered will be.
Everything you dream will become true.
Everything is possible you will see.
Your family united we will see you succeed.
Everything you do, do it with love.
Keep the good and pure saved in your soul.
Always moving forward courageous and strong.
Everything will come in life. God bless you, my love.

You are the crown of your grandparents,
and your talents are precious treasures.
More than a brother more than a friend,
you are our inspiration my lovely son.

Keep the faith, forgiveness and love,
the compassion happiness and hope.

Everything you touch prospered will be.

3. I want you to know ... I'm unique, do not compare me

"... Grandparents, uncles, neighbors, teachers I like to be the way I am, I am nice and affectionate, kind and polite, hardworking and funny. God made me unique, just like you. When you compare me between your grandchildren and compare my failures with the successes of others, I do not know what to do. You do not see me or what I am, but you see autism and that is like a ghost in your eyes that does not let you accept me as I am. I have a unique personality just like you and talents to succeed in life, just like you. I need only one opportunity to be myself and do not compare me with others, I am Unique and Original ..."

Have you ever had the feeling that your child is different? Or that he does not behave like the children of your friends or family? Where do these thoughts come from? You have probably been comparing your family with other people's families, but you should not feel bad, because this happens to everyone, even to excellent mothers like you. They are simply biological and social instincts that are rooted in primitive thoughts of social hierarchy.

The comparison is the process through which we examine two or more things, with the sole purpose of establishing differences or similarities between them. Comparing is part of our daily life, this helps us make decisions and assess areas of everyday life. In some cases, we usually compare our houses; or perhaps our cars, with those of the people of our social circle, only to see what position we occupy in the hierarchy of society, but sometimes it is not necessary to establish certain comparisons; as it is in the case of our children.

Comparing our children with other children, most of the time, is not a good idea nor is it appropriate. Because when we compare our children with those of our neighbor, our co-worker or simply the children of our brothers, we can affect, and even unnecessarily hurt, the feelings of our child, since he will wonder if there is something wrong with him or if he is different, this unnecessary comparison is directly affecting his self-esteem and his identity.

Sometimes, there are cases where some parents are discouraged to see that a child has an extraordinary talent and your child does not have any, do not fall into envy. This happens because they are constantly making comparisons between their kids and other people.

It is very important that you always have a positive mind, it is much better to see the glass half full, to see it half empty. In life always will be presented people with successes above or below us. There will always be someone with better or worse abilities, but the important thing is to recognize that we are all good for something and that we have a reason to exist, a definite and unique purpose.

Each child, during his own development, is showing the diverse abilities that God gave him, and is our own job as parents to discover them and to help our children to develop their talents to the fullest, with lot of love, patience perseverance and hard work. It is important that you focus on the progress your child is making, and that you reinforce it by helping him to continue working to fulfill his goals every day.

How can you help your child to develop his talents?

29

MY SON, what every child with Autism wants you to know

1- Identify the potential of your little one. You should look at what are the interests that your child enjoys; as well as in what kind of activities does it work best for him. Obviously you must think about both, the preference of your child and what makes him happy, as well as what he does well and naturally perform with excellence. All people have even one talent, and it is your job and responsibility to help your child discover and develop it , since this talent he has may be enough to create a future life, with victories, happiness and fulfillment.

2- Celebrate the effort and not the qualifications. You must encourage your children that it is important that in each activity they perform they give one hundred percent of themselves. It is important that we as parents celebrate the fact of seeing our children working hard to complete a task. However small it may be, from the first words, to when they recite the alphabet for the first time. Even if they are wrong, it is important that they feel support, and that they learn what effort is more effort; it is equal to excellence, regardless of the setbacks or mistakes they have had, they will always serve as teaching to succeed.

3- Reinforce originality. After you have discovered the talent that your child has, help him believe that it is wonderful and that makes it unique and different from others. It does not matter if he plays the piano, and another child can also do it, the simple fact that he plays it, makes an extraordinary and unique task. Focus on valuing and startling that originality of your child and reinforces positively, with gestures of love; as hugs and kisses, each of his talents. Reinforcing his originality, you will build a beautiful and indestructible self-love and high self-esteem, which will help your child grow happy and complete.

4- Perfect His skills. If you already discovered for what activity your son was born, or what his natural ability is, as for example; you heard him singing a song and you noticed that he has a very beautiful and well-tuned voice, now it's your turn to help him perfect that skill, so that one day the fruit of all his efforts will be to reach a professional level and be able to live from his talent.

Each person has a unique, exclusive dream inside their heart. So, together with your child it is our job as family to help the new generation to discover what they are passionate about,

MY SON, what every child with Autism wants you to know

so that they achieve success in their lives and develop those talents to the fullest potential. In the near future they can fully develop what their really love and have a life full of happiness and prosperity. Of course, there is no hard work when you do what you love and have passion for it and you can live from that.

Conclusion, the comparison only exists in order to overcome or be better than another person, but if that other does not exist, neither does the comparison. Focus on competing with yourself, because the only barriers between you and success are in your mind. Get better every day, and it becomes the best version that can exist of yourself, and most importantly, encourages your children this way of thinking. Some children will be the next architects, carpenters, farmers, presidents, dancers ... billions of professions that will be given in relation to their talents and abilities, we are all different and we do not deserve to be compared with anyone.

The road to success is paved from failure to failure. Try your best! Until you achieve it. **Yes, YOU CAN DEFEAT AUTISM! Read up to the end!**

4. I want you to know ... I love to take a ride in mom's car

"... I am neither a motorist nor autistic (as some people call me). My name is not autistic, nor is my profession autistic. I'm David, I'm a writer and musician, that autistic thing was invented by the devil and I do not allow you to call me that name, ever. I am the blue-eyed boy with a mother full of faith and a loving and playful Dad. Could a health condition change my name? I remind you, David Perez, the Rubio Perez, the champion of mom and dad, that's me. Do we understand each other?

I am David, son of God, chosen between ten thousand with destiny and eternal purpose, head and no tail, blessed on coming and going and everything that touches my hands will prosper. My mom wrote me a song "My Son" with those words, to remind me that I am David, the treasure of Mommy and Daddy ... "Yeah! and I love riding in a car, like all children does.

Traveling in a car or moving from anywhere can be seen as something usual and common; but still driving on the road, traffic and rush hours in the city center promote stress to all of us. Children have a limited patience and tolerance than adults have. When they get bored on a trip they tend to get irritable; endure the trip sometimes is frustrating for them. Safety when traveling in car is a very important issue for both children and adults.

The mandatory use of the seatbelt is a current traffic standard in all countries of the world. Many accidents and tragedies have been avoided or could have been avoided by complying with this requirement to use the seatbelt while driving. It is a behavior that we must inculcate to all the members of our family.

In particular families that have special people, the use the seat belt inside the vehicle while driving is paramount.

My son takes off his seat belt while driving and we almost have an accident

It is an experience that mothers with special children live on a daily basis. Security is important and not just for us; but also for other people who travels on the roads. It is always better to be safe than be sorry.

1. Prepare a schedule;

with your appointments, another for your partner's appointments and one for your children's schedule. With that schedule you can better organize your time and the time of everyone else. You can be ready for any unexpected incident. Your structure and organization will provide the flow of the activities of each member of your family and home fluency. You will be able to handle the situations that could appear, and be safe when your child removes the seatbelt while riding in your car.

2. Invest time training everyone;

Children and adults learn by imitation and repetition. Teach them from the first time to use the safety belt; make them understand what it is for and how it works. Train them before leaving on a trip and they will have practiced correctly as well as putting on their belts; Keep it on for the entire duration of the trip. Remember that it is not to have him imprisoned, suffocated and immobile.

3. Bring a cooperative companion;

MY SON, what every child with Autism wants you to know

it is a good idea, that the companion is ready to help and pays attention to your children while you are driving. You need someone to sit in the back sits next to them, so that if something goes wrong, they can help the child at the right time.

It is also a good idea that your companion takes turns with you to drive the car. At some point of the trip, the child will need assistance and your peer can give him 100% of the attention, in order to be calm and you can still drive the car. It is not recommendable to stop the car in the middle of the road because you are alone and in charge of everything and that may cause an accident and is even a dangerous situation.

Always stop in safe areas if you need to and call 911. Is non useful taking a companion who does not cooperate during the trip, and who is on his mobile and distracting the situation talking to you and making you nervous.

4. Carry variety of accessories;

they work well to distract your child's attention, so you keep it attached to the seatbelt. There are infinities of inventions created for this purpose, nor can you imagine the variety; you can search them on the Internet, they are accessories that are put on the seat belt.

These accessories prevent the child from loosening the belt unexpectedly while driving the car. All these accessories are tested by experts in security systems. You cannot invent and improvise on your own, which could then endanger your safety, the safety of your children and other drivers who circulate at the same time as you on the road.

5. Communicate with people who already have experience;

it is always good to seek help, advice and communicate your needs to other mothers who, like you, have special children. They will give you ideas of how they solved their security situations while driving in the company of their children.

6. Use an additional rearview mirror;

You can use an additional rearview mirror to look exclusively at the child. It is useful to look back from time to time when driving; so you check if your child is well placed, with his belt and has no signs of boredom. Always have both hands on the wheel.

7. Keep toys handy; we know that every special child has his favorite objects and toys: key chains, anti-stress ball, stuffed animal, his favorite blanket, etc. When you go in a trip, I recommend that among the things you prepare for the road, include a bag with these preferred items of his choice.

Sometimes the stressful situations that happen inside the car happen because your son does not know what to do, while you are driving the car. Place the bag of toys next to you, that you can offer your child different entertainment options while you drive the car. I recommend to do so while you stop at the light.

8. Do not talk on the phone while driving;

this is one of the laws that all drivers must obey in general. In many countries the use of telephones while driving is prohibited. The telephone is a great communication tool; but driving a car at same time you use your phone could become a fatal trigger.

Do not send text messages or talk when you drive. If you need to know an address where you are going, prepare in advance the GPS of the car before leaving. It will be activated without needing you to touch the phone. It also prevents you from taking the wrong way. Remember always to be calm if you lost the way and return by the right road.

9. Keep your hands free; at all times.

Have your hands free, do not occupy them with the telephone and keep them always on the steering wheel while you are driving the car. The security of all depends on how committed you are to work with this situation, we know that it is not easy.

Turn any car trip into a fun and safe time. Mom, you are the one who knows your child best and the reactions he has to different scenarios; you know what he needs and wants; Take advantage of your knowledge about his preferences.

It is good to have extra support; you are not alone in this mission. Remember your family is special and you are special too.

MY SON, what every child with Autism wants you to know

Yes, YOU CAN DEFEAT AUTISM!

Read up to the end!

5. I want you to know ... Can you help me to wait for my turn?

Oh no! that line is so long! I get bored when I have to wait a lot in the same place. I do not know where my body is and then I move it a lot to feel it. I do not do it on purpose, I cannot control it, they all look at me and look at my mom and even they get mad on her, they say that I'm not well educated. It seems they were never children before, and if they knew how hard it is for me to overcome autism every second of my life, they would help me make the wait more fun or let my Mom go first. She is my hero; she always manages to leave me standing with honor in front of the whole community.

Being in public places, where the flow of people is intense and constant, is cumbersome for children with autism. My son was always very anxious, and showed frustration to be in places with strangers for a long time. Whether we were in line to pay at the supermarket, in the doctor's waiting room, or in congestion in the car, it was difficult to get David to be calm and safe.

MY SON, what every child with Autism wants you to know

After a while dealing with this, I learned how to successfully handle these scenarios, and you as a parent must also do so. The first thing is that you should not feel ashamed of your child, even if he makes tantrums in public or starts to getting upset, and all people are looking at you with rarity judging you wrongly. People always looks astonish when these situations happens, and first-time parents who have not yet learned how to deal with autism, cause a feeling of strangeness.

Do not limit and deprive yourself and your son to go anywhere and always you and your family is locked up at the house because you do not like to go out with him. Your son deserves that you, as parents and family, want to take him everywhere, because you feel proud and happy that they see you with him.

rom going out to have an ice cream, going to the movies, the supermarket or to the Church, you must teach your son how to appropriately behave in these places, and you must learn how to handle the tantrums and also have patience with others who do not know how to help you. Talk with the specialists, who are treating your son, to give your ideas or also that the specialist accompanies you to that specific appointment as part of your child's recovery and the effective integration of your child and your family to the community.

Many times there are very kind and respectful people near you who do not dare to help you if you do not ask them. That is why a good attitude and communication with your neighborhood will help to make the long wait easier. Long waits are tedious for you, so for a child with autism, it is more.

I know you've noticed that your child becomes frustrated, in these scenarios, and because they do not like to wait. It disorients them to not be able to do anything for a long time, and more if you are scolding them at every moment, so that they are still. Scolding and calls for attention do not usually result in any child much less with those who are overcoming autism.

It is best to teach them appropriate strategies to entertain them and to entertain themselves adequately wherever they go.

1. Patience

The essential thing is that you have patience, because your child feels how you feel. There is an emotional connection between parents and child, so as you feel your child will transmit it, he will also feel what you transmit. If you get stressed, he will get more anxious.

Learn to be patient, if you are not calm in situations where your child is upset, you will never manage the situation. You should always have a smile on your face and treat your child always with love. Remember that you are also in a public place, where everyone observes how you deal with your child. **The soft response appeases anger.** People are cruel, they laugh or they are afraid or they do not know how to help you. For that you must prove to yourself, your child and others, that you are able to handle the situation calmly, be patient. Show that calm, love and patience to your child, this way you will feel calmer. **Effective and calm communication is the key.**

Plan and Organize.

You have to think about all the situations that could arise, on the street or on the trip. Maybe your little one is hungry, wants to play, he evacuated in his diapers, has dirty clothes, and many other things. It is recommended that you bring with a bag, where you get everything you need. Start with basic things, and then go stuffing things for emergency.

Basic things to carry in your bag.

✓   • Whole foods, fruits or snacks. It takes several options because the craving of your child can be very selective or special food according to your child's diet.

✓   Milk or milkshakes, juice and water.

✓   • Toys, sensory toys from which he chews, toys those he interacted with. But be careful, do not take the whole house with you. Take those light weight things to carry easily.

✓   • Medicines. He may have a fever, or he may hurt. So it is good to prevent, if you were on vacation or a trip of many days.

✓   • Clothing. Maybe he starts waning because it's cold or hot, or he gets upset and he wants his own flannel. Also he got his clothes dirty while eating, and wants to change his clothes. Always preventing a tantrum is wise.

✓   • Towel, wipes, antibacterial lotion, diapers and soiled diaper's bags. While waiting in line, this can happen. And the correct thing is that you change his soiled diaper in private and return to you place in line.

MY SON, what every child with Autism wants you to know

You have to be prepared mentally and materially, to solve all problems. The most difficult problem that can be presented to you is a diaper change while you are waiting in line. Do not cry, this happens to anyone and is normal. People around you may bother or express their discomfort. Your reaction should be quick, with a big smile asking for permission to change your child in the bathroom, quickly do it and then come back.

Do not apologize, because there is nothing to forgive, people must learn to be tolerant.

3. Another difficult situation, is that your little boy during a tantrum, will hurt another person or is aggressive. It does not usually happen as much, because children who have symptoms of autism as we know, do not like to interact with other people and hurt himself instead others. But if when they get upset and become aggressive, be patient and talk calmly and ask for help.

It is a very delicate situation; to which you must have an incredible wisdom There are sympathetic people, like others who do not. So always be as polite as possible, and if you have to apologize for the discomfort, just do it. Remember that you represent your child, and everything your child does, you have to be responsible for.

Always schedule all the trips you will take with your child. Think of all the scenarios that can be presented to you in that place, and you are prepared for everything. So that you do not forget, write in advance everything you need in a book, and hours before leaving prepare everything. Do not leave anything for last.

Finally, if it is the first time you will leaving your house and you are very nervous.

4. Recreate the trip at your own home. You can do a simulation, of the waiting room or the row you will take, or in the street, and have your child participate, to see how he behaves. In this way you will know what to expect when you leave your house, and how to deal with any complications. Always have a good attitude of learning and reinforce your child with words of love all his effort even if it is minimal. Ask for ideas and strategies to specialists and talk to friends who have overcome long waits.

Yes, YOU CAN DEFEAT AUTISM!

Read up to the end!

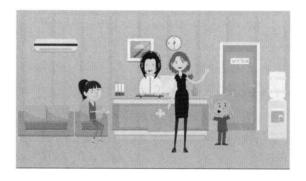

6. I want you to know ... I need help to organize my playing time

"... It fascinates me, it talks to me all the time and it answers me every time I touch it. The lights, the sound and the vibrations of the IPad are my obsession. But I like better the affection of my family and my friends. Do not leave me alone with the IPad and send me to I pad's jail that I do not know how to get out by myself. I need you..."

Another concern that parents have with children with autism is how to make our children's day to day productive and rich. I got a question from a very worried mother, where she said that her son spent all day in the IPad and what she could do to end this repetitive behavior and obsession. Removing an object from a child who has symptoms of autism that is entertaining him and is their favorite toy, is an emotional shock for them, so they tend to get upset and very angry escalating at levels that could be uncontrollable and dangerous. That also happens with adults and anyone.

MY SON, what every child with Autism wants you to know

Technology, in these times, helps us a lot with our children education, but it can also be our worst enemy if we do not know how to control its use. Technology in these times is not only a tool to help the human being, in some cases it is also a tool for addiction difficult to overcome. It is sad to see how even at home, communication and interaction are lost, just because each member of the family is in their own virtual world. But this can be worked and fixed. Downtime or leisure time is dangerous!

Down time or free time is dangerous!

Imagine if already for an adult it is difficult to control the use of his virtual technological devices, is worst for an innocent child. The addiction to technology arises from the dead times that people have. A person with a lot of free time at home, who has access to the Internet and a Tablet, will spend all day stuck and trap there. For our children who have a lot of free time, because they are almost always at home, it is very easy for them to get addicted to social networks. So we as parents must avoid this at all costs and dose and organize exposure to empty technology time.

For a child who has symptoms of autism using technological devices such as the Tablet, it is great because they could be educational or communication tools, but always with control and adult supervision.

The children are very attracted to the complexity of the device and the automatic sensory response from it. All children always demanding for a lot of attention and the device is giving the attention you don't, so they want to use these artifacts more and more for being so flashy, so imagine and so close to them. The main idea is not that you totally forbid or prevent your child from using technology, the main idea is that you control the time on the device and you are responsible and must decide the timing of each thing that helps better your child.

You have the responsibility to organize your child's daily routine. You must make a rich and varied itinerary, of the activities that you will do every day, during each hour and each minute of his daily routine. **Plan your child's day 24 hours, so that he always has something to do, productive and educational and not fall into a down time.**

MY SON, what every child with Autism wants you to know

With a good plan that you fulfill to the letter, I assure you that your child will be able to achieve it and will not even think about technological devices or video games.

What we want to achieve with this, is that the child is always entertained and producing life and never get bored or empty or dead time. You have to convert every day of your child, on productive days.

The good side of technology: Your child can use technology in a productive way to achieve progress or to communicate. There are many software and equipment that are special for children with autism and other medical situations, so these must always be the goals of your child. If you have a Tablet, delete and block all applications that you know are not aged appropriate and only leave activated for use those that are educational for your child.

You can also use the IPad as a motivation to work as a reinforcement for your child's effort. Example if your child does not like it when he is going to receive his educational lessons, and he always gets frustrated with the class, you can start using it as a motivation or reward. Show your child that if he behaves well and does his homework, he can use the IPad for a short period of time.

Do the same technique with adults in the home, lest you be addicted to the internet and the child is just imitating what you do. If you see symptoms of addiction to technology, please seek urgent professional help.

Learn how to educate your child, because he has autism, does not mean he will always do what he wants. He is a child as the others, who needs his parents to teach and put limits. But with limits I do not mean scolding, scolding promote more rebelliousness in children with symptoms of autism and in general. **Always avoid aggressive talking and punishment,** you must find a nice way to correct the weak areas of your child. As parents it is not easy to deal with all this, because you see how your nephews with only one warning they listen, and your son is not like that. Love your child and love your life, never covet your child to be like another child, give thanks to God for him.

Be the Role model of your son!

MY SON, what every child with Autism wants you to know

Maybe you think that because your child has a medical situation he is not following your example and role model. **Remember the children are the reflection of their parents**, so you have to start with yourself. It's ironic that bothers you that your son is always on the IPad, and you do the same. Before we bother with someone about something, we must evaluate ourselves, and think about whether we have the right to get angry. It would be very unfair for you to scold a child for doing something that you also do. Take the iPad out of your life, and out of his.

Decrease the use of devices of everyone's life at you home. it's time that all that time your child is investing on the IPad be invest on a fun activity. Look for something to do productive for him and for yourself. Well, you will not remove the IPad to leave it with dead time again, because it will always return to it if you don replace it with something else.

✓ **Mom, I want to play!** Here are a few suggestions of activities that your child can do in his daily routine. Introduce different activities to the daily routine so they are no so repetitive over and over the same game.

Remember that you should start doing these activities with him, and then leave him by itself once in a while so that he becomes independent and familiar.

✓ **Finger Paints:** This is a very economical activity, as simple as some construction paper and a few tubes of finger paints. This activity can entertain your child for a while. Always all activities must be with adult supervision. In addition, he will develop his artistic and imaginative play. Remember that around the activity is the entire organization of the materials, collect, clean, select. Write a small agenda with activities related to the selected game

✓ **Toy box.** A play area where he plays and find toys, is very good because all his concentration will be on toys, games and educational activities. Choosing toys for educational and sensory purposes will give a better acceptance and recreational input.

• **Sing and dance.** A musical space is great to have at home to motivate your child. Music is always a good therapy for everyone. Set up a music area in the living room with lively music, and close to your child sing and dance. We always recommend that you do activities with your child and closely supervise them. Prevent your child from taking toys to his mouth or using them inappropriately. That will be a challenge that you will face and train your child to appropriate play is very important.

Physical activities and sports, Walking, running, cycling, kicking a ball, swimming, jumping on a trampoline, horseback riding are activities that not only distress anyone but also have other developmental, sensory and neurological benefits.

Yes, YOU CAN DEFEAT AUTISM!

Read up to the end!

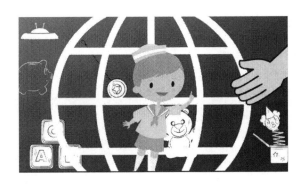

7. I want you to know ... I like family vacations

"... I can hear the comments of mom and dad, worried about how the family, which is supposed to accept me as I am and cooperate with my recovery, will react when we go on vacation. In those days all my skills and situations are exposed and Mommy and Daddy 's work is to give me a decent life. I smile at everyone with my best smile, but how it hurts when they ignore me and judge me for my health ..."

Go on vacation with the family, it is a topic that extremely worries any parent. The thoughts of being away from home, which is the environment where your child develops daily, and go for many days to a new place is to sit and think. The anxiety to try new things is something normal in the human being, but in children with autism it intensifies a thousand times more. If in the car sometimes your little child does not behave very well, surely you do not even want to think about how he will do it on a plane.

MY SON, what every child with Autism wants you to know

Do not discard the idea of traveling, or spend a nice vacation with your family for which they will say. Although it is a little harder to travel with your son, you will see that when the trip is over, it will have been worthy the effort. There is nothing more beautiful, than being next to the people that you love most, sharing new adventures. Besides that, this retreat will suit your child very well. For always being at home, or frequenting the same places always, they bore and can even depress. Taking a family trip adventure is always fun. All your family already accepts your little boy and they love him, so everyone must support and help each other, to make the trip they so desire.

Planning My Vacation with My Family

For the grandma who asked me the question, you can start by talking well with your grandchild's mother. And this goes for all the grandmothers who read me, the support of their grandchild's parents is the first thing to look for this holiday. In this way, together with them, they can plan and organize the trip, since their parents know everything that is needed and required to make this long-awaited trip successful.

Taking into account the fact that each of the family members should be more than willing to help in any unforeseen situation, I will give you below the following tips that will help you give your special grandchild such a vacation that they deserve so much.

Planning My Vacation with My Family

For the grandma who asked me the question, you can start by talking well with your grandchild's mother. And this goes for all the grandmothers who read me, the support of their grandchild's parents is the first thing to look for this holiday. In this way, together with them, they can plan and organize the trip, since their parents know everything that is needed and required to make this long-awaited trip successful.

Taking into account the fact that each of the family members should be more than willing to help in any unforeseen situation, I will give you below the following tips that will help you give your special grandchild such a vacation that they deserve so much.

1-Plan the length. Better is short trip and good, than long and boring. On your grandchild's first vacation, it is important that is for a short period of time; like one or two days. And it is important that they are relaxed during all this time of travel, since sometimes we have so many expectations, that most of the time some of the goals are not reachable due to factors related to the same time or external.

2- **Find a neutral place.** The place chosen for the holidays should please both children and adults; So that each member of the family enjoys this time outside of the routine. They can be places like the beach or some places outside with fresh air, where children can relax in a park and adults can have fun while supervising them and being safe. It is important that children have personalized activities with professionals, because if your grandchild gets bored there could be room for unpleasant situations.

3- **Easily Adapts to changes.** When you leave the routine for the first time, a little anxiety always appears, especially for your grandchild. You must be mentally prepared for any kind of inconvenience and changes, and have a plan how you would solve that situation. When we talk about holidays, anything could happen, an activity could be canceled and your plans change, but you should remember that the most important part of the vacation is to create a pleasant atmosphere and strengthen the bond of love with your grandchild. A good attitude at all times will help to have a great time. Leave aside your personal demands and cooperate with this unique opportunity. Try not to talk frustrated in front of your grandchild because he understands your emotions and his esteem could be affected.

4- **Always supervise your children.** Sometimes we go on vacation like going to the grandmother's house and we forget that we have a child with special needs and we want the child to adjust to our life as the elderly. We must always be available to help our grandchild, as we must also have the help of another family member to take care of him and make sure we are always there for him on the trip.

You must leave leisure and technology for a while, and concentrate on this special time, which will be short, but invaluable.

5-Ignore the offenses. During the travel you have seen many different people who do not know your situation. It is important that you are emotionally prepared to overlook any kind of offense that may trigger some kind of fight or confrontation. Have a good attitude always friendly and polite, do not make faces or speak from behind. It is very ugly that the family of the special child is the one who criticizes and judges the most.

The most important of all is that you enjoy every single detail of the trip, do not wait to get to the destination to start enjoying your grandchild. Since the memories of the preparation, and even those of the road are some of the best moments which you will never be able to forget.

The healthy love of the grandparents is irreplaceable in the life of any child.

Yes, YOU CAN DEFEAT AUTISM!

Read up to the end!

8. I want you to know ... I am part of your family, accept me as I am

"... I did not choose you as a family, I did not ask to be born. Autism does not interest me at all. Some people loves me and others not so much. I am a gift from God for the one who receives me and the one who rejects me loses the opportunity to receive my pure, faithful and sincere love. I am gentle and gentleman of good taste I am the happy child the champion of the house as my mother calls me ..."

When a baby is born, from the first moments of his life he has a desire to communicate. They are interested in the faces and images they see on a daily basis and try to understand everything they see.

The everyday faces that surround them and the activities that happen motivate them to participate even before they emit sounds or say a word.

During the first years of a child's life, motivation must be given to develop their language and to teach them to speak.

In some cases, with special children it is a little more complicated due to this condition that affects communication.

MY SON, what every child with Autism wants you to know

They have difficulty communicating with the environment because autism affects part of their abilities and development. As a parent, grandparents or relative of a person with special conditions is normal that you are worried about being able to effectively communicate with your child but it is not impossible.

Signs of autism:

✓ **Lack of Communication:** Within the forms of communication, which are presented in the signs of autism there are too many. Well, several of the communication skills could be affected and each child always tries to express himself in his own way. But nevertheless, we can generalize some, and from there start to solutions. We have to be responsible, the ones that first in helping our children to improve communication. Therapies doctors and teachers will help and train you, but you have to incorporate and generalize that learning into real life.

• **Non-verbal.** When you see that your little boy, he is already 2 years old and still says nothing, not even "mom", or any word at all, is that he could present this type of autism's sign. You could think that he was even speechless or deaf, but you saw that when he does a tantrum, he screams loud. He does not say words, but he does make sounds. This is one of the most common signs for autism, and the most difficult to deal with.

Nothing is impossible for the one who believes. Love, will be your gasoline and motivation to defeat autism, never get discouraged, even if you see other children younger than your child that said "mom" and "dad". The love covers a multitude of lacks.

The love and acceptance you give to your child give him the security and support he needs to overcome autism. The more you delay to do something about the speech the more he will regress in his language.

The speech pathologist will help you do certain communication exercises to achieve and recover the ability to talk. Every sound counts, every gesture counts. Do not underestimate your child's effort to communicate.

✓   • **Echolalia.**

MY SON, what every child with Autism wants you to know

This is happening when your child has already shown you that he can say whole sentences, but when it comes to a long conversation, is difficult to sustain it. Instead of continuing the conversation with you he repeats whatever you said or ask. One of the most common examples is that you ask your child "How are you?", And he will respond "How are you?". This means, that he repeats things, and having difficulty to make the effort to formulate an answer to it. A lot of people will think that your son is making fun of you but is not. Think about autism effects in communication and affecting the way processing the language to have an immediate response, so repetition is what you will received as an answer.

Spontaneity. It is when the child is struggling to overcome autism and only has one topic of conversation. Something that he is passionate about and cannot stop talking about it. For example, your little boy arrives and he starts talking about cooking toast. But then, he ends up talking about a magical world where the toasts are wonderful. When you notice this, rejoice that your child is a few steps away from fully overcoming autism and with exercises you can train the child to respond with various topics and discuss other topics as well.

You are the center of your child's progress, if you wait for the specialist to do everything for your son, the advances will be few. A specialist teaches your child, words, phrases and complete sentences, the basic, so that he understands a little, how to react to possible scenarios. Now it's up to you as parent, the hardest part, to give the confidence and motivation to generalize communicate and socialize, both with the family and outside the home.

A grandmother asked me how I can help my grandson to talk and here are some suggestions for family members.

1. Establish emotional acceptance: accept the health condition of your family member as it is. Speak to your grandchild with love, if you find yourself away for some reason or you live away or in another country; you can send letters, gifts, and voice messages over the phone. They have to know that they are loved and accepted as they are, how they are and what they can give at this time.

It is truly important for them to be accepted and not be rejected, so they will not be inhibited from wanting to speak and express themselves. Many times people who have health conditions or physical impairments, in addition to feeling bad about this, are judged, rejected, discriminated against, ignored. The worst thing you can do with a special person is to ignore it, in doing so you reject it and they realize this. They recognize the people who accept them and relate positive relationships with them.

2. Establish eye contact; the eyes are very important in any type of communication. Look closely into the eyes of your son or grandchild. In some therapies for example, the specialist puts something striking between the eyebrows (a very interesting idea): a cookie, a sticker, the favorite toy to capture the attention of the child's eyes and keep watching. When the child responds by watching intently, fuss over him, congratulate him because he is making a great effort when looking into his eyes, something extremely important. You cannot establish an effective language if there is no visual contact. Eye contact is the first form of communication between two people; the first thing we do is to look.

3. Respond to any gesture; It is not necessarily to answer with words. The child can respond with a hug, with a gesture, raising his hand. They respond even with small grimaces with their mouths, sometimes imperceptible for the development of a talk, the greatness of communication. With all this they are saying something. The non-verbal message is very important, because before speaking they will try to communicate in their ways, not verbally and this is also a communication language.

4. Wait for the answer; many times we get involved in repeating and repeating sentences and we do not give the child time to react and respond. A hello, hello, hello hurried and repeated stuns them; we do not let him respond with a hello, with a raised hand. Give him the opportunity to answer, and vary the phrases you use to address him. And wait for the answer for about 5 or 7 seconds and then ask again. If the third time you ask after waiting for the answer does not respond, then give the example how to respond and practice it with him.

MY SON, what every child with Autism wants you to know

Yes, YOU CAN DEFEAT AUTISM!

Read up to the end!

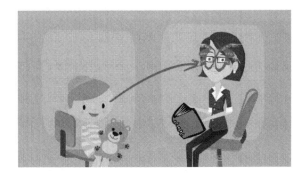

9. I want you to know ... I love to walk on tiptoe

"... I'm a genius and I love heights. Mom, I do not feel my feet, but when I stand on my toes, that pressure on my fingers is an extraordinary sensation that's why I do it all day long. It is not funny not to feel your body, to want to run and the body walks. I love the massages on the feet and my mom says that I frame the rhythm of the music very well. Can you help me use my body properly without judging my movements?

Autism is a condition characterized by presenting a series of signs in various areas of behavior such as repetitive and stereotyped movements. Maybe your little boy makes stereotyped repetitive movements, which you think are normal, that get your attention and you scold him for that and his little brothers but the behavior goes on and on. And the truth is that it could be the common signs of this childhood syndrome commonly called autism.

Many parents are living with the confusion of noticing this signs for autism on the behavior of their children, and those that are their commons behaviors. Because it may also be that your son is behaving badly with his little brothers, but you for having patience for his condition do not take action on the matter.

It is not wrong to get confused, because any parent who does not know about autism can do it. Before I was in the same position as you, but that did not depress me, instead I urge to be more knowledgeable about the subject and how to help my son. This is the purpose of this book, to give you information so that you are alert and help your children to overcome autism at an early age.

How to Identify the Signs of Autism?

A mother asked me a question, very puzzled and worried, about her daughter walking on tiptoe every day, all day long. Previously I had already commented, that this is a typical sign of autism, and the children find it more interesting to walk like this. We already identified several features of autism, but now I want to dive deep into the subject.

Well, before I get deep into the subject so that you would realize that your little boy could had autism now I am showing you that you can learn about the behaviors, gestures and actions that you can expect from your son.

Most of all I want to talk about stereotyped movements, which tend to be very repetitive and rigid. Although each person is different, autism has the same pattern that occurs in all people who are affected by this syndrome.

• Patterns

One of the things you will notice the most, is the rigidity of the movements and behaviors. They tend to spend all day, doing the same thing. Example: sat on the floor to play with a car, and spend 5 hours and still in the same place with the same position. If he is lying down, he wants to lie down all day. If you woke up walking on tiptoe, you will do it all day long. It's completely normal for them, because children who have symptoms of autism when they get comfort in something, last a long time enjoying it.

This is not the only way you will see in automatic behaviors, but you can also get used to sitting in the same dining room chair every day, or on the same side of the furniture or just like to sleep with a sheet and see only one television channel. The patterns are also very remarkable, such as listening to songs in the order of the alphabet, or using their crayons to order colors in the rainbow. In communication you can notice, that he spends a whole day talking about a single topic, no matter how hard you try to change it. Finally, it may be engaged in only one part of the toy, Example: your little girl plays with the Barbie but the only thing she does all day is to turn the little arm.

Beware of these patterns and your way of trying to modify them, because when he establishes a repetitive pattern, or he gets used to doing something in a way, and a day comes when he does not do it, he can form tantrums and big tantrums. Even physical aggressions you can receive, on the part of your son, thus removing him from his routine is a great emotional shock for him. But as a good parent you are, I know that you will have all the patience, love, consideration and dedication to help you get out of the stereotyped patterns and redirect to appropriate and productive movements for the child and always try new things. The behavior therapist (ABA) is responsible for training your child and the whole family to know how to deal with these automatic and repetitive stereotyped movements.

✓ **DON'T PUNISH! Redirect Some mothers,** relatives or educators punish their children for these automatic movements and even put them in times out. BAD! VERY BAD! These stereotyped movements are involuntary and above there are ignorant people who punish children for that. Punishment only brings more problems,

STOP! so please train yourself educate yourself and get out of ignorance. Special children are people, human beings and should be treated with love professionalism and patience. I suffered a lot with my son with non sensitive educators who put my son in penitence for stereotyped behavior, What sadness! and shame others give me that finds people in educational positions doing such kind of thing.

FLAPPING HANDS

In the gestures we could include, what a mother told me that her daughter did a lot. Walking on tiptoe is one of the most common sign of autism. Another thing they do is make gestures of wings like butterflies with their hands, or raise and lower their arms. They may spend all 3 hours playing this way, as it may be that it is quite small and make this gesture spontaneously. This is stimulation or self-stimulation, which is the same. Because touching his eyes or ears for a long time is a sign that this stimulates him, and seeks to feel that way.

✓ **SENSORIAL STIMULATIONS!**

Through the repetitive gestures your child makes, he stimulates himself. It may be that your child looks at things, touch things, smell things or try things. All this because he is discovering little by little how to get stimulation. It may be that he claps for 30 minutes, because he likes the itching on the palms of his hands. Or that he smells your hair for a long time, because he loves the perfume of your shampoo.

Beware of stimulations because they can lead to accidents, there are children who sadly find stimulation by biting themselves, so take care of your little one from this. Redirect that behavior with something more productive.

✓ As he grows up you will know what stimulates your little boy, and so you can take advantage of this and stimulate yourself.

This way you will be able to strengthen the father and son bond, which is so important to us parents. The idea is that you play a lot with him, and stimulate him, not that you try to remove the gestures that he likes. Clear everything in the picture, that this does not affect him in anything bad, or those around him.

Stimulation is very important for our children, because it helps them overcome the limitations of autism.

✓ **Transitions**

It is when you go from one place to another, and this causes an emotional shock. For example: you may plan to go to the park and he is refused to leave the house. It makes you all a tantrum but you manage to get it out of the house, get to the park and calm down quickly. And so the time goes by all right in the park, until it's time to leave and this makes another tantrum. These moments are called transition and you must learn how to handle it.

For that you will create a visual agenda on a paper or on your phone or on your IPad where the child knows what will happen next and you anticipate talking to him with love and showing him photographs of what he will do in the other place.

Many times these tantrums occur because they do not want to leave what they know for the unknown or think that there will be no food or games that they like. So talk to your child as much as you can and even if you do not receive an answer from your him, do as if he were answering you. He will feel safe to go from your hand and always inspire confidence that everything will be good fun and will return home in a short time. You can also show him a watch to tell him how long they will be in that place and why and then he can return to his comfort zone.

Communicate. Use all kinds of communication with your child, visual, gestures, auditory, sensory. Always speaks with him normally. You will see that in the future he will thank you for giving him the opportunity to integrate normally into your life.

Do not leave anything for granted, communicate with the child as if he understood everything. Of course, special children have more developed senses and can perceive your emotions and decode them. It seems ironic that a child who can barely speak is much more sensitive than someone who seems to talk a lot. The brain is receiving all the information and you will see the answers very soon. So always keep a good positive attitude and faith in front of your champion.

Yes, YOU CAN DEFEAT AUTISM!

Read up to the end!

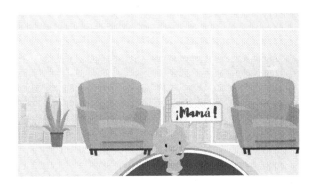

10. I want you to know ... What makes music to my brain

"... I am a musician and a writer as my mother. Music is one of my favorite communication languages. Every time I play the piano I feel complete, successful. Although I do not understand well what I sing I remember all the lyrics of the songs and I can write them on my IPad. Do we sing together?

The last tool that I want to give you in this book, so that with your help and God's help, your child overcomes autism, is music. We have to have faith in all the tools that we have, and the ones we can provide to our children. Do not give up or faint, God is with you, and I am with you, so you are not alone

Throughout my life, I have always liked to try many things. Well, because I had my son David with autism, I was motivated to find ways to help him. But one of the things, which I did in my life without knowing that later it would help me so much with my son, was to teach music since I was 12 years old. I played the piano since I have memory use, and that helped me from an early age to be able to teach music to others.

MY SON, what every child with Autism wants you to know

What I liked most about all this, was teaching children the art of singing, in the choirs. It was so long ago, but it served me as my experience, so that the idea of "piano-therapy" was born, which is what I am currently working on. There are parents who call "music therapy" others piano-therapy, the things is that any therapy with music helps people who are going through a difficult time, or situation that involves their health to improve. Through the years I've been teaching music, I've seen the great help that music does, and how important it is in the life of a human being.

Lalaland, autism is over.

Music helps, as big as you can imagine, to children who are affected by autism, or any other neurological disorder, because music stimulates the entire brain. The advantages, benefits and pros that you can give to music, with respect to what it does to your brain are many. Everything is because nothing else can stimulate the brain so completely and intensely. The simplest and best way to stimulate, the brain of your child is through music. None of the neurological stimulating machines, with just a few minutes of music per day, make a great impact on your child's life.

Anyone likes to listen to music, their brain works just like everyone else's. The brain moves trying to process everything that music means.

Think about this, the music not only implies to understand the lyrics, but to enter in tune with the beat. They are all parts of your brain working together, focused on one thing: music. The purpose of doing music is to find pleasure in it.

I know that the children I help with "music therapy" could learn more than a song in the day. Your brain learns unconsciously to archive, organize, add, subtract, combine, identify, among other things. All for a simple rhyme. This is a way you cannot forget this tool, will help you to help your child and overcome autism. What I do ask you is that you take it seriously learning music as your reading or math classes. Do not see music as an alternative, supplement, fun or extracurricular activity. You have to see it as something serious and important, could be your child is a musician and will have progress and overcome autism with this talent.

Mom, I want to be a MUSICIAN!

MY SON, what every child with Autism wants you to know

It is not only that your little boy listens to music, it is that he also starts playing an instrument. Because it is not only to enjoy music, but also to be part of it, it will increase the levels at which music makes your brain work. The things you will learn without realizing, when learning to play an instrument will be many, that even you will be surprised of the advance.

Just like when your body thanks you for exercising in a gym, and you start releasing toxins out of your body, so will your child grateful for playing and instrument. His brain will start to work more, compare to anything else he does, because the music serves as an alarm for the brain and awakes those parts of the brain that autism puts at rest or blocks.

Music requires discipline and perseverance; it must become a daily routine for your child. The more professional you are accustomed to being, the better the results will be. He has to enjoy the moment, because what we want is a good neurological stimulation with joy. The brain gear benefits more and more, when the child repeats the action of playing the instrument until the piece is perfected. In all disciplines, perseverance is the key to success.

It is scientifically proven that counting or reading produces a brain stimulation of the size of a grain of salt, compared to the size of the brain stimulation produced by playing or producing music as the size of the world.

• **Inappropriate behavior.** The cries, screams, blows and tantrums will diminish, so that it is rare whenever you see it. Good behaviors and good manners improve, and even repetitive gestures that you know are not right, will disappear little by little. The child will develop his talent and this will level the other areas that are weaker.

My experience with music and autism: My son David.

Of course I included my little son David, in the piano-therapy, and hey, he's the best example I can talk about, like I know that music works. He has already learned to read music, to play piano and to listen to it, in a way that you would not think is a child that has symptoms of autism. You as parent should not limit your child, because he is capable of everything you believe. I already have students, who made their own mini orchestra, and present themselves at their school, concerts and are professionals.

MY SON, what every child with Autism wants you to know

Did you see everything that music does in our children? I recommend that your child have at least 4 lessons per week for music classes, and that he learns to play the instrument that he likes the most.

Yes, YOU CAN DEFEAT AUTISM!

Read up to the end!

Conclusion

God's plans for our life are perfect and pleasant, and I hope that when you undertake the long journey you will realize it. In same cases dealing with autism is not that difficult, as people who do not know about it paint it. It's all in the attention that you give to your little boy, because if you fill him with rejection, hatred, and stress, he will rather sink into autism more and more.

Those parents who live stressed, who hate having a child with autism, and who treat their children all the time with screams, only retract and grow the neurological problem that is affecting their children. This is how autism wins, and the child becomes violent and very rebellious. You have to find an engine that motivates you every day, be a better parent for your little boy.

Love is what should always be, because if you do not transmit that to your child nobody will. If you start accepting your child and loving him as he is, your family and close friends will also do so. Acceptance is the most important step, in the goal of helping your child overcome autism. Your focus should always be that, in overcoming autism, but without falling into despair and denial that you are going to "fix your child." Well, he is not damaged, only that he neurologically presents a disorder that you can help recover. Never let someone else make you think otherwise, or let you choose between your child and her or him, because if a friend does not feel comfortable with your child, then you do not need it in your life.

Remember that your child should always be your priority, if you wanted to have a child so much that autism does not making you no longer want him. Autism is just one of those challenges that life puts you, and that you must confront and emerge victorious from it. Remember how David beat the giant, when everyone thought it was impossible. You must be a David for your child, and beat autism regardless of whether everyone shows a negative response to it. Everything happens for a reason and there is a purpose in it, and who are we to discuss decisions to the King of Kings and Lord of Lords.

I hope that at the end of the book, if you felt anxious about the situations generated by autism, you will not feel that way anymore and get up to work. Your child needs you and you are the person chosen and best selected to help him. That you feel like helping your child, and coping with the situation is the best idea you can have, start now. Remember that in this you are not alone. First you have God, who has created us with all the love of the world and you have yourself and you have your son. Without God we are nothing, so cling to your faith in God and make it your rock of support, because nobody will help you like Him and HE will give you the comfort you need.

This book was born with the idea of helping parents and families get up and understand that having a child with a medical condition is not a bad thing to die regardless of the medical situation. Turning pain into a gift and seeing the smile of many children and families is the purpose of this book full of love, passion, compassion, patience, experiences, laughter, tears, experiences and professionalism. I even thought that God was not fair and he had forgotten about me and I asked myself why me? I came to the darkest depression and the feeling of guilt chased me day and night.

Remember that your child should always be your priority, if you wanted to have a child so much that autism does not making you no longer want him. Autism is just one of those challenges that life puts you, and that you must confront and emerge victorious from it. Remember how David beat the giant, when everyone thought it was impossible. You must be a David for your child, and beat autism regardless of whether everyone shows a negative response to it. Everything happens for a reason and there is a purpose in it, and who are we to discuss decisions to the King of Kings and Lord of Lords.

I hope that at the end of the book, if you felt anxious about the situations generated by autism, you will not feel that way anymore and get up to work. Your child needs you and you are the person chosen and best selected to help him. That you feel like helping your child, and coping with the situation is the best idea you can have, start now. Remember that in this you are not alone. First you have God, who has created us with all the love of the world and you have yourself and you have your son. Without God we are nothing, so cling to your faith in God and make it your rock of support, because nobody will help you like Him and HE will give you the comfort you need.

This book was born with the idea of helping parents and families get up and understand that having a child with a medical condition is not a bad thing to die regardless of the health situation. Turning pain into a gift and seeing the smile of many children and families is the purpose of this book full of love, passion, compassion, patience, experiences, laughter, tears, experiences and professionalism. I even thought that God was not fair and he had forgotten about me and I asked myself why me? I came to the darkest depression and the feeling of guilt chased me day and night.

I was able to get up and help my prince overcome autism. I am passionate about his progress, his unique personality, his unparalleled smile, his love without words. My vision changed, instead of seeing what was missing I learned to reinforce what I had, to see his abilities instead of his limitations. I learned that my life was not the same without my little angel David. He taught us true love, without words or glances, he gave a special meaning to my life and changed the whole family. It is the most beautiful and beautiful thing that God could have given us.

MY SON, what every child with Autism wants you to know

I was chosen among many women as the best and only qualified for this possible mission and to be the mother of a champion. I was selected from the specialized squad of great challenges and my beloved son gave me the opportunity to grow and to love unconditionally.

I have more than 35 years of experience teaching music to children, two university degrees, one in music and one in theology, 12 books written music productions, radio TV programs, I have traveled almost all the continents of the world and taken my musical message to all nations. I am a woman of faith, successful and hardworking. Autism changed my life and my priorities and I do not change professional success and all the money in the world for my family. My family is my priority and my son my mission.

I want to extend my helping hand so that through this book you receive answers, tools and faith. I want you to also see your champion achieving his purpose in life and that you are special. Finally, you have your family, who will give you all the physical and earthly support you need.

No one said it would be easy, nobody said it would be simple, but that's what we are here for, to learn to be what someone thought impossible, possible. What is impossible for men is possible for God. God bless you always, and fill you with blessings. Come on and Get UP You can do it!

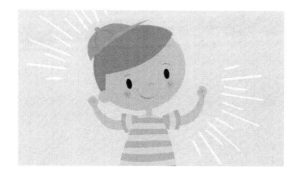

Yes, YOU CAN DEFEAT AUTISM!

Read up to the end!

BIOGRAFIA: LICENCIADA SILVANA ARMENTANO

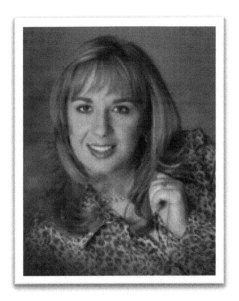 Silvana Armentano Pérez: Mom, wife and friend she is a producer of radio and TV, music, composer, writer and piano teacher composition and voice, currently lives with her husband Daniel Pérez and his son David Pérez in Florida, United States. Silvana teaches and trains musicians from around the world. She began her career as a piano teacher in Argentina at the age of 12.

She graduated with a Bachelor of Music at the Conservatorio de Música López Buchardo in Argentina and revalidated her degree at the University of Miami, United States. She studied composition at UCLA and studied piano and singing with different recognized teachers and vocal trainers. She also has a Masters in Theology and has written a number of books of faith. She won several awards for her compositions and participated in the OTI Festival, San Remo and Latin Grammy's with her own songs and musical productions. She also has more than 12 books written and 13 albums of Christian music recordings and 5 productions in secular music. She has also written a series of articles for different magazines throughout her artistic career. Her passion as a teacher is to discover the talent of each student and train them to be a professional and happy musician. Through overcoming autism every day at home she learned a new language of communication and teaching strategies through music.

She currently receives training in Autism along with his son, more than 50 hours per week. With these tools, they have been able to communicate effectively with each child for their talents and abilities and to get the precious diamond that is in them regardless of their medical situation. She looks at her students with passion, vision and love and coach them to give them a tool in life to defend themselves, live from their talents and be happy. Silvana has more than 35 years of experience teaching music to children and adults of all abilities and her entire life as a musician. She is the founder of Musik Hope, a non-profit organization, whose vision is to develop all children

MY SON, what every child with Autism wants you to know

focusing on their talent and musical ability. Musik Hope purpose also is to aims to bring information and awareness about this childhood syndrome called autism, for parents, family members, teachers, leading educators, pastors and the community in general. Persistence, professionalism, love and vision are some of the characteristics of this mission to develop the musical and artistic talents of each student and each family has the necessary tools to help them overcome autism.

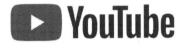 Subscribe: Silvanaarmentano

CONGRATULATIONS YOU ARRIVED AT THE END!

YOU CAN OVERCOME AUTISM!

ORDERS, INVITATIONS, Conferences,

CLASSES and Interviews

Visit My web Page:

silvanaarmentano.com/MUSIKHOPE

Or Call 786-558-3777

More information:

musikhope4kids@gmail.com

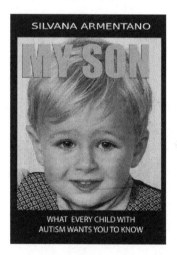

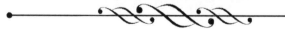

Made in the USA
Middletown, DE
14 January 2020